KETOGENIC DIET

How I Lost 60 lb in 6 months

ASIF IQBAL

HEALTH DISCLAIMER

This book provides general information and discussions about health and related subjects. The information and other content provided in this book, or in any linked materials, are not intended and should not be construed as medical advice, nor is the information a substitute for professional medical expertise or treatment. The opinions and views expressed on this book and website have no relation to those of any academic, hospital, health practice or other institution.

"Without your health, you've got nothing going on. I thank God every day for good health." Ric Flair

Table of contents

1) How I lost 60 pounds

2) What I Ate
    a) Breakfast
    b) Lunch
    c) Dinner
    d) Drinks
    e) Snacks
    f) Desserts & Natural Sweeteners

3) Foods I Avoided - Kryptonites!

4) Fasting Fast Lane

5) Exercise Smart

6) Sleep Better

7) Avoid Loose Skin

8) What's Next

9) FREE Gift

Book Resources

Go to
https://asifim.com/keto

- Grocery List
    - Walmart List
    - Amazon List
    - Dirty Dozens to avoid

- Smart Kitchen Essentials that makes your life easy
    - Blender
    - Indoor Grill
    - Food Processor
    - Air Fryer

- Supplements

- Best home scale and exercise equipments

"Without your health, you've got nothing going on. I thank God every day for good health." Ric Flair

1. HOW I LOST 60 POUNDS

My weight loss journey started back in 2017. I was 60 pounds overweight, had high blood pressure, and lived with all sorts of pain—knee pain, back pain, you name it. I didn't sleep well most nights and I felt heavy and lethargic during the day. I was the posterboy for being fat and sick.

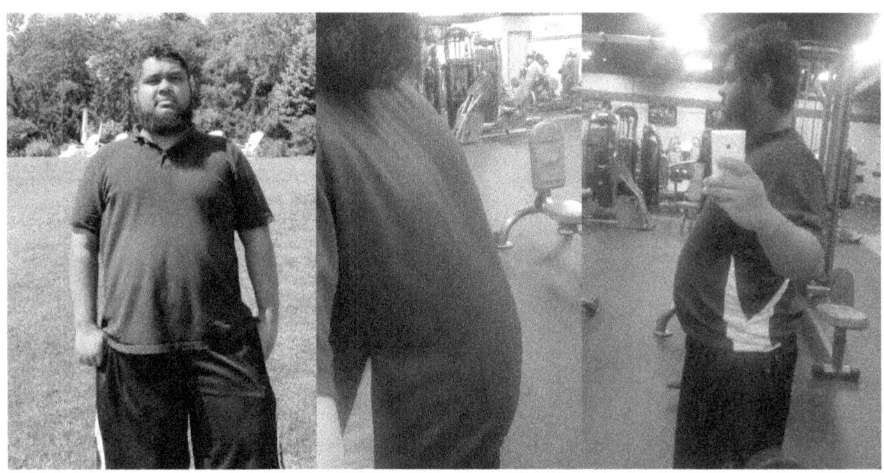

I was so unhealthy that although I was living the entrepreneurial lifestyle I had dreamed of—making money online while I slept and having the freedom to work from anywhere in the world—I was hiding behind a penname online, afraid that people wouldn't take me or my business seriously if they knew how I'd let myself go. Honestly, I was so embarrassed of my weight that I never posted any full body photos on Facebook, and even went as far as avoiding visiting my family for a few years. I felt like that big of a failure. The shame was as crushing as my ballooning belly.

Then, in mid-2017, I met Dr. Nevada Gray, who introduced me to living a ketogenic lifestyle and taught me some serious exercise hacks to get my health and life back. As I applied what I learned, the pounds started falling off. The chronic pain faded and I began feeling like myself again. I slept better and had energy like I'd had back in high school! I was finally able to enjoy the time, freedom, and money I was earning from my online business, travel without any health issues to hold me back, and confidently rekindle relationships with my friends and family. Things turned around, all thanks to going keto.

The goal of this guide is to share how I lost 60 pounds and got my life back. I'll be sharing the exact blueprint that made the magic happen. It can work for you too, if you're willing to give it a try.

Enough about me; let's get straight to the good stuff. If, like me, you can't stand reading fluff, here are the Cliff Notes of my journey:

"Without your health, you've got nothing going on. I thank God every day for good health." Ric Flair

Summary of How I Lost 60 Pounds

- Ate a "ketogenic diet" which was about 75% fat, 20% protein, 5% carbs
- Enjoyed customized meals that are healthy AND tasty, while avoiding all foods that can cause inflammation (check out my keto cookbook if you want to see the flavorful, easy-to-make meals I created)
- Started working out 20 minutes a day, eventually increasing workout time to 60 minutes within 6 months
- Drank lots of water, lemon water, apple cider vinegar with water and green tea.
- Intermittent Fasting - ate my first meal at noon, my second meal by 6pm, then nothing until noon the next day (18 hours)
- Slept 8 quality hours each night
- Took natural supplements to increase results (like garlic and turmeric)
- Consumed collagen through bone broth or supplements to reduce likeliness of loose skin and stretch marks

If you're interested to know exactly how you can lose weight, end your aches and pains, and feel young again, grab a cup of coffee and read this short guide till the end. I will share all the secrets I learned so you can live your best life, too!

"Money doesn't mean anything to me. I've made a lot of money, but I want to enjoy life and not stress myself building my bank account. I give lots away and live simply, mostly out of a suitcase in hotels. We all know that good health is much more important."
- Keanu Reeves

"Without your health, you've got nothing going on. I thank God every day for good health." Ric Flair

2. WHAT I ATE

A. BREAKFAST

Until I discovered the benefits of intermittent fasting and fasted cardio (more on those later), I was drinking bulletproof coffee for breakfast. It's a great way to jump start your morning with a boost of healthy fat. You'll stay full longer and have laser sharp focus.

Here's a typical morning:

1. Right after I woke up, before anything else, I drank 3 to 4 cups of water. I added ¼ of a freshly squeezed lemon or 1 tablespoon of Bragg's Organic Apple Cider Vinegar to a cup of water.
2. I drank bulletproof coffee after 1 hour. Followed this basic recipe:
   - 1 cup brewed coffee
   - 1 tablespoon of salted Kerrygold Irish butter
   - 1 tablespoon MCT oil
3. Went to the gym for 15 minutes (increased it to 30, 45 and 60 minutes in few months).
4. Drank more water, 1 to 2 cups at least

There is nothing wrong with these steps if you are an

absolute beginner in the ketogenic world. Once you get used to this lifestyle, I suggest you look into the benefits of intermittent fasting, which we will cover in Chapter 4.

You will learn that the best breakfast is no breakfast (you still drink 3 to 4 glasses of water, though). Skipping breakfast and exercising in a fasted state will result in maximum weight loss. But again, this is not for absolute beginners! Take it slow and ease yourself into the lifestyle. You'll be surprised at how quickly you start losing weight even when you're starting with the basics.

B. LUNCH

Soup & Salad are the simplest and most practical lunch, in my opinion. And trust me, these aren't light pickings; they're full of the fats you'll need to stay satiated. To make it even easier, I prep my salad ingredients twice a week, on Sundays and Wednesdays, and prepare homemade broth once a week, on Sundays.

I'd suggest eating organic whenever possible, or at least avoid produce in the dirty dozen (*Go to asifim.com/keto for Book Resources*). Adding a few spoonfuls of high-quality cold-pressed extra virgin olive oil to your salad or soup will help you reach that

70-80% fat calories ratio.

I find it helpful to eat lunch around the same time each day, between 12 and 1pm. Remember to drink more water before and after, about 1 liter (4 cups) if you can.

It's best not to drink water 30 to 45 min before or after a meal so it doesn't dilute your stomach acid. We want to be able to digest food as effectively as possible and absorb maximum nutrients.

Salad:

I mix and match the following as they are on the safe list according to most experts I follow:
Romaine Lettuce, Cucumber, Red Cabbage, Avocado, Red Onion, Red Radish

Dressing:

Raw high-quality olive oil, avocado oil, or Primal Kitchen Avocado-based dressing or Mayonnaise, lemon juice, Himalayan pink salt or homemade vinaigrette

Bone Broth Soup with Himalayan Pink Salt:

Chicken, beef or goat bones cooked in a large slow cooker for 24 hours (yes, it really takes that long to get all the beneficial collagen and other nutrients into your soup). Add water until bones are just covered. I often add veggies at the end (such as cauliflower and broccoli) and extra Himalayan pink salt before drinking it. Check the resources section if you want my exact recipe. This makes about a one-week supply.

Consider taking a 15 to 30 min walk during your lunch break. It can give you an energy boost when afternoon fog tends to set in.

C. DINNER

Dinner is the best time to be creative and try out different recipes. Here are my general guidelines to come up with a perfect ketogenic dinner:

1. **Fat**: avocado, ghee, raw olive oil, raw coconut oil, avocado oil, pasture-raised eggs, beef/duck fat (e.g. leftover fat from beef bacon)
2. **Protein**: Palm-sized, one-inch-thick fish (wild-caught preferably) or cage-free chicken or grass-fed beef/goat/lamb
3. **Veggies**: lots of veggies, like half of your plate. This is easy to measure; just take one to three handfuls of veggies. I eat a lot of broccoli, mushrooms, red onion, cauliflower (I especially it like shredded/riced), asparagus, spinach, kale, french-cut green beans, brussel sprouts, okra,

sauerkraut

Remember, a ketogenic diet is a high fat diet, not high protein. Choose fatty cuts of meat or fatty fish, such as salmon with skin on. Don't be shy to eat more eggs (best if high-quality & pasture-raised). Add raw olive oil or cook with ghee or beef bacon fat.

Check out the 2nd book in the series, Ketogenic Cookbook, for breakfast, lunch and dinner ideas.

D. DRINKS

While on this diet, I only drank the following drinks, which have zero net carbs.
Net carbs (digestible carbs) = total carbs - fiber.

Sticking to these drinks will help you lose the most weight.

- Water
- Sparkling Water (unsweetened)
- Lemon Water
- Apple Cider Vinegar mixed with water
- Homemade Natural "Gatorade" (see resource for recipe)
- Herbal Tea (see grocery section for a full list)

- Green Tea
- Black Coffee

After I lost 60 pounds, during the maintenance phase, I added the following drinks, which are low carb.

- 100% pure coconut water (imported from Thailand)
- Fresh vegetable juice
- Coconut milk (unsweetened)
- Flaxseed milk (unsweetened)
- Cashew milk (unsweetened)
- Almond milk (unsweetened)

"Without your health, you've got nothing going on. I thank God every day for good health." Ric Flair

E. SNACKS

Snacking in general is not a good idea, so I tried to avoid it as much as possible. If you have to indulge, the best snacks on a ketogenic diet are fat bombs, which is just a cute nickname for high-fat foods. There are many recipes for fat bombs but this is one of the easiest to make and my personal favorite.

Two ingredient chocolate fat bomb:

- 1 cup extra virgin coconut oil
- ½ cup cacao powder

Slightly warm the coconut oil. I like to microwave it for 30 sec in a microwave-safe dish. Then, slowly mix the cacao powder into the oil, one spoon at a time. Pour the mixture in a silicone chocolate mould (available on Amazon). Last, freeze them for 1 hour and they should be ready to munch on. Be sure to store them in the fridge as they will melt at room temperature.

F. DESSERTS & SWEETENERS

On a keto diet, I had to be careful not to overdo desserts or sweet drinks. Even though you can sweeten foods with natural sweeteners, which are zero carb, natural sweeteners can still cause insulin spikes, which will derail your weight loss.

For the bakers out there, here are the top ketogenic flours:

- Almond Flour is high in fat, low in carbs, and moderate in protein. It is more dense than coconut flour and is usually a 1:1 substitute for regular flour, unlike coconut flour.
- Coconut Flour is very high in fiber and low in carbohydrates so it is perfect to use in baked goods such as breads and desserts. Since it is high in fiber, it usually only requires about 1/4 the amount of substituting in place of normal flour or almond flour.

These are cornstarch alternatives, for when you need to thicken your food:

- Glucomannan powder
- Almond flour
- Ground flaxseed

"Without your health, you've got nothing going on. I thank God every day for good health." Ric Flair

- Chia seed
- Mashed cauliflower

Some natural sweeteners (use sparingly):

- Erythritol Powder
- Monk Fruit Powder
- Stevia Powder
- Stevia Liquid

3. FOODS I AVOIDED- KRYPTONITES!

It's equally important to know what foods you should avoid when you go keto. If you've done some research, you may have noticed that every health expert has a slightly different list of no-go foods. This is because some are more strict than the others. It's best to be a little disciplined in the beginning if you want to lose weight quickly. Following a ketogenic diet for weight loss is most effective, in my experience, when you avoid all types of simple carbs and any foods that may cause allergies or inflammation, like dairy products or artificial sweeteners.

Low-Quality Oil

Avoid all types of low-quality oil such as vegetable oil, canola oil, corn oil. They aren't the heart-healthy fats we want to load up on.

Artificial Sweeteners

Avoid all artificial sweeteners, such as aspartame, which is present in most diet soft drinks and sugar-free gums.

"Without your health, you've got nothing going on. I thank God every day for good health." Ric Flair

Processed Food/Fast Food

I avoided all foods that contain sugar, rice, wheat, i.e. processed food or fast food.

Nightshade Plants

I avoided nightshade plants (tomatoes, eggplant, peppers, chillies etc). But it's up to you if you wanna be that strict. There is a debate among some doctors that they can cause inflammation.

Raw Foods Containing Oxalic Acid

I also avoided eating some food raw. Foods which contain oxalic acid, include leafy greens like spinach, kale, chard, parsley, collards, and beet greens. Spinach has the highest levels of oxalic acid – 750 milligrams per 100 grams serving. Feel free to eat them cooked, just not raw.

Farm-Raised Fish, Poultry and Eggs

I avoided all types of farm-raised seafood, such as tilapia, shrimp, catfish etc

4. FASTING FAST LANE

So far, we've touched on the basics of a ketogenic diet. If you follow those, you should be golden, but if you're itching to lose weight even more quickly while resetting your body's functions, my tip for taking your weight loss to the next level is adding a few different fasting techniques. You can try them all or choose one that fits your lifestyle.

FASTING IS ONE OF THE MOST POWERFUL WEIGHT LOSS TOOLS.

If you're taking notes, write that big and bold. Fasting makes you eat fewer meals and can lead to an automatic reduction in calorie intake. It also brings a sense of discipline to your diet routine.

A. INTERMITTENT FASTING

Beginners 16:8 Fasting

This is the easiest way to start. You'll eat 3 meals a day within an 8 hour window and fast for 16 hours. So let's say you:

- Eat first meal at 8am
- Eat second meal at 12pm and
- Eat third meal at 4pm

Then, approximately 4pm to next day at 8am, you eat zero calories, only consuming water, tea or other zero calorie drinks. You'll have fasted for 16 hours, which might sound like a lot, but you'll end up sleeping most of it. Getting started is the most intimidating part.

Intermediate 18:6 or 20:4 fasting

This method of fasting allows for 2 meals a day within a 4 to 6 hour window, so you fast for 18 to 20 hours, depending on when you eat your first meal. So let's say you:

- Skip breakfast and workout in a fasted state
- Eat first meal between 12 and 2pm and
- Eat second meal before 6pm

Then, from 6pm to the next day at 12 or 2pm, you eat zero calories, again, only drinking water, tea or zero calorie beverages. It sounds tough, but as always, I suggest easing into it by taking your time before you move onto more complex forms of fasting. Listen to your body and do what works for you. You may be surprised at how refreshed you feel after a few days.

Advanced 22:2 fasting or One Meal A Day (OMAD)

This is only for advanced dieters. You eat everything within a 1 to 2 hour window, meaning you eat one meal a day and fast the rest of the time. So you:

- Skip breakfast
- Skip lunch
- Eat first meal between 4 to 6pm

Then, from 6pm to next day at 4pm, you eat zero calories while making sure you have lots of water, tea or zero calorie drinks. That's a 22-23 hour fast! It's pretty intense so this is definitely not something to jump into without experience, but it can be an amazing way to lose weight and rejuvenate your system.

B. BONE BROTH FASTING

This is my absolute favorite type of fasting. I usually start it on a Friday so it ends on a Sunday. If you want to look 5 to 10 years younger and fix your gut health, look no further. For 3 to 7 days, I drink bone broth and around 2 liters of water per day. That's all. You might be thinking, no meals?! Yes, no meals, but bone broth is known as liquid gold for a reason. It's full of nutrients, fulfilling fats, a high amount of collagen and really nourishes your gut. When doing a bone broth fast, I'm even able to go to the gym and do all my regular exercises.

C. WATER FASTING

I tried water fasting for 3 days. This is only for super advanced dieters. It has a lot of health benefits when done properly. Here are a few tips I can give you from my experience:

- Do it during the weekend or a time when you can relax at home
- Expect dizziness and headaches
- Mix Himalayan pink salt, potassium salt, and baking soda with water to replace electrolytes

- The doctor I follow suggested not to overdrink water (2 liters or 8 cups is enough)
- You might lose some muscle mass
- In 3 days, expect to lose 3 to 5 pounds

"Without your health, you've got nothing going on. I thank God every day for good health." Ric Flair

5. EXERCISE SMART

If you are an absolute beginner, remember that 5 minutes of high speed walking is better than no exercise. I have friends in wheelchairs, and some of the only exercise they can do is wheel themselves around. They give their best effort, despite their handicap situation. If your legs are working, be grateful and use them more often!

I got gym memberships to my local Planet Fitness and YMCA. You don't necessarily have to have a gym membership, although I'd highly recommend it. Any physical activity like swimming, biking, playing tennis, football, or cricket is equally great - just do what you love! Move around as much as possible and be active. Maybe go to the mall or your favorite park to get started.

My typical gym workout:

1. One mile elliptical
2. Five to ten minutes treadmill at 3+ mph. If you are overweight, I do not recommend running. It can give you knee and ankle pain.
3. Machine weight exercises (rather than free weights as this is safer for beginners)

4. Stretching & physiotherapy exercises

"Reading is to the mind what exercise is to the body."

- Joseph Addison

"To enjoy the glow of good health, you must exercise."

- Gene Tunney

"Few people know how to take a walk. The qualifications are endurance, plain clothes, old shoes, an eye for nature, good humor, vast curiosity, good speech, good silence and nothing too much."

- Ralph Waldo Emerson

"Without your health, you've got nothing going on. I thank God every day for good health." Ric Flair

6. SLEEP BETTER

Back before I started keto, I would snore all night and keep everyone up - there are so many embarrassing stories about that lol. I used to wake up every now and then due to breathing issues. I also had inflammation and pain, which often stopped me from falling asleep or made it impossible to reach deep sleep. On a keto diet, I found it was much easier to sleep well at night.

After diet, sleep is the 2nd most important factor in weight loss and getting healthy. You might be surprised that many experts consider it more important than exercise! There is simply no alternative to a good night sleep. I have done some extensive research on sleep by reading books and hacks by Tim Ferris, Shawn Stevenson (author of Sleep Smarter) and Dave Asprey (founder of the Bulletproof Diet). Here is a summary of my research:

- **The most important thing is the mindset that a good night sleep is gold; it's priceless and something no amount of money can replace.**
- 10pm to 2am - these 4 hours are the best time to sleep according to much scientific research.
- Drink caffeine only during breakfast or lunch time (before 2pm).

- Soak yourself with enough sunlight during the day to reset your internal sleep clock (AKA your circadian rhythms)
- Magnesium is great for relaxing the muscles. You can take it in many ways - Epsom salt bath, Magnesium Oil spray or Magnesium Tablet supplements
- Take a natural supplement such as Melatonin (start with 1 to 3mg) or Valerian Root tea or capsules. After taking it, turn off all lights, otherwise this won't work.
- Do not use bright white lights in your bedroom after evening. That includes your phone, tablet, laptop, or TV screen. It mimics sunlight. Use apps such as Flux or iPhone's built in feature to reduce white light if you have to use your devices late into the night.
- Do high intensity exercise everyday, even if it's just 15 minutes of high speed walking. In other words, do exercise that will get your blood pumping.
- Stop drinking water a few hours before bedtime so you don't have the urge to pee in the middle of the night.
- Gut health is super important for a great night sleep. Drink your homemade broth everyday. If you feel hungry at night, don't be shy to drink

another cup and add some himalayan pink salt.

- For pain and inflammation, take natural supplements such as MSM, Turmeric and ginger capsules.
- Use a body pillow to avoid low back pain.
- Invest in a good quality pillow. Experiment with a few brands and find one that suits you.
- Many sleep experts say sleep temperature is important for a good night sleep. Best is not too hot and not too cold, somewhere between 60 and 67 degrees Fahrenheit (16 to 20 degrees Celsius)
- Last but not least, get used to a firm bed. Soft beds might be comfortable but is it good for your back? Trust me, you will get used to it in a month.

7. AVOID LOOSE SKIN

The ketogenic diet is one of the best diets to make you look younger and feel better at the same time. It has the potential for rapid weight loss, which seems like an ideal thing, but this can also lead to loose, flabby skin and extreme stretch marks. There are even TV shows about how people lose huge amounts of weight and then have to deal with these unwanted side effects. Most of the time, people turn to surgery, but that's expensive and risky. That's not an option I'm willing to consider, so I did a lot of research into alternative methods for avoiding this problem.

There are two main secrets to avoid skin-tightening surgeries:

1. Eat a high fat diet rich in collagen, which will improve skin elasticity. Fill your body with collagen, amino acids and other nutrients by drinking 2 to 3 cups of homemade bone broth. Take collagen supplements if you need to.
2. Do some arm and ab exercises everyday to tighten up. They are the most common areas to get loose skin, so do more abs crunches and lift more dumbbells or kettlebells.

Tips: Do these everyday and you will not only lose a lot of weight but have a great looking body too.

"Without your health, you've got nothing going on. I thank God every day for good health." Ric Flair

8. What's next?

Now that you are equipped with the exact same blueprint that has helped me lose 60 pounds, it's your turn to take action and make it happen. In a few weeks you will see great results and you will thank yourself!

Go to asifim.com/keto for all the book resources.

Before you go grocery shopping, go through your section of kitchen cupboards and fridge. Anything that's not healthy doesn't belong there. Donate it or give it to a friend. That my friend is the #1 step you can take right now!

Definitely checkout by 2nd book in the series - Ketogenic Cookbook, where I will simplify some of the most scrumptious recipes I have seen in the keto world with easy to follow instructions.

"In the midst of these hard times it is our good health and good sleep that are enjoyable."
- Knute Nelson

9. FREE Gift

If this book inspired or motivated you, please give me a review on Amazon and send me a screenshot to comtechmn@gmail.com. I will personally reply to your email with my top 10 dinner recipes!

*"Help others and give something back.
I guarantee you will discover that
while public service improves the lives
and the world around you,
its greatest reward
is the enrichment
and new meaning
it will bring to your own life."*

Arnold Schwarzenegger

*"Without your health, you've got nothing going on.
I thank God every day for good health." Ric Flair*

www.ingramcontent.com/pod-product-compliance
Lightning Source LLC
Chambersburg PA
CBHW061326250726
48657CB00003B/1069